Profitable
Niches
in
General Dentistry

Profitable Niches in General Dentistry
for
New Patients
and
Practice Growth

Amol Nirgudkar, CPA, CGMA

Profitable Niches in General Dentistry

ISBN: 0615893112
ISBN-13: 9780615893112
Library of Congress Control Number: 2013917534
Amol Nirgudkar, CPA, CGMA, Tampa, FL

Published by:
Amol Nirgudkar, CPA, CGMA
13940 N Dale Mabry Hwy, Tampa, FL 33618
www.reliancecpa.com

813-931-7258

First Edition (February 14, 2014)
Printed in the United States of America.

*Dedicated to helping dentists
develop the profitable practices
of their dreams.*

Don't sit down and wait
for the opportunities to come.
Get up and make them!
—C. J. Walker

Contents

Introduction

Why place focus on developing a dental practice niche?

As professionals, we devote a substantial portion of our lives toward becoming skilled at the art that we choose as our career. We strive to become technical experts in our field of expertise and aim to serve our clients to the best of our abilities. Implicit in our hard work is the desire to be rewarded for our skills and dedication to our field. Additionally, over and above the mental satisfaction of serving our clients, we all seek to maximize our financial rewards. Our ultimate objective is to enjoy practicing our art and gain financial freedom and independence.

For most of us, financial freedom can be achieved through higher earnings during our working years. Achieving the goal of financial independence within this time constraint necessitates an efficient allocation of our priorities. Maximizing our earning potential every day will help us attain true financial freedom.

So how can a dentist earn enough to enjoy financial freedom and independence? How can a dentist maximize daily earning potential? You could simply work eighteen-hour days, but this option doesn't leave you much time to enjoy life outside the office. Additionally, depending on how you manage your practice, working longer, harder hours won't necessarily yield the most economically optimal outcomes. How you use your available time on a daily or even hourly basis can optimize your earnings-to-working ratio while enabling you to maintain that all-important balance between work and life.

In the dental industry, we've seen an influx of special services that general dentists can offer patients. More so than ever, general practitioners are choosing to diversify their practice by offering specialized services. With one-visit procedures, fast orthodontics, cosmetic smile makeovers, sedation dentistry, snoring and sleep apnea appliances, temporomandibular disorder (TMD) therapy, headache solutions, immediate dentures, and amazing new technology, general dentists can now provide their patients with expedient, expert care for a range of health concerns. Most of these innovative treatments do not require specialist training, though certification and continuing education are required or recommended for some.

In this book, you'll learn how developing a niche can:

- Supplement revenues and enhance profitability.
- Provide patients with a one-stop customer experience.
- Position you as the local expert ("artisan dentist") in your niche area of expertise.
- Bring your dental practice targeted cases for optimal success.

We will take you through the evolution of a niche practice from conception to successful execution and enhanced profits. You don't have to come to the table with experience in market research and sales. This book will be your guide through all aspects of building a niche dental practice, so you can focus on your patients and practice, instead of spending countless hours at business seminars. Additionally, the book will end with marketing ideas that are relevant and important today.

The epilogue will introduce a brand new system of dental marketing that will set your practice on a phenomenal growth trajectory. During the course of my decade of consulting, many marketing concepts have made the rounds through my office. Some were absolutely brilliant, and others were complete gimmicks. The DR.4 system is a crystallization of all the ideas that have worked and proven to be successful in the professional marketing space.

The DR.4 system that I have developed is a holistic approach to dental marketing focusing on the four *R*'s of dental marketing. A system that will **Reach** the right patients, enhance your **Reputation**, foster sophisticated and targeted patient **Reengagement**, and finally create a plethora of **Referral** opportunities.

Are you ready to explore the road to success? Your journey begins here.

Chapter One: Planning for Success

*By failing to prepare,
you are preparing to fail.*
*—Benjamin Franklin,
America's original entrepreneur*

We get paid for bringing value to the marketplace.
—Jim Rohn, American entrepreneur

Determining Your Niche

Market Research

You learned it in school: the rule of supply and demand. Before any business launches, its founders should study their audience to determine if the demand for their service or product exists. This is particularly true of companies, like dental practices, that serve clients in a specific geographic region.

Demographics

The term *demographic* refers to the characteristics of a particular group of people. In marketing, important characteristics that define a demographic include:

- Gender
- Age
- Family size
- Race
- Income
- Values

You may at first think that some of these factors are insignificant. For instance, your practice caters to men and women of all ages, races, and incomes. While that may be true, the demographics of your community

will help you determine whether a particular dental niche might succeed
or fail.

Know Your Demographics

Most dentists cater to patients who live within twelve to twenty miles of
their office. Sure, you may have clients who fly in from Europe, but for sheer
economic reasons, the great majority of your patients will live near your
practice. *In most cases, the female in a household selects the dentist for her
family or boyfriend.* These characteristics are true for most dentists, so
we'll assume they're on target for your practice as well.

When it comes to market research, you need to understand the people,
particularly women, within twelve to twenty miles of your practice. You
should know where they work (if they work), where they go on weekdays and
weekends, and what type of social activities they enjoy. In addition, you must
understand their finances, values, and life goals. Know where they live and
where they vacation, shop, and congregate.

To run a successful dental practice, you have to serve your patients' needs,
tailoring your services to who they are and where they are. Will your niche
service meet their needs or accomplish their goals?

A family dentist in a suburb of Houston caters to a wide range of demographics. He decides to focus on implant dentistry, with the goal of attracting
more implant patients. He has taken advanced courses and seminars on the
subject and is well trained in treatment by equilibration, orthodontics, and
oral splints. He adds a page to his website describing his service and publish-
es an ad in a regional magazine. He invests in developing a logo, signage, and
a micro-website about implants. Would he be successful?

During the same time period, a general dentist who primarily serves adults
in metropolitan Seattle adds an implant niche to his practice. He, too, has
significant training in implants. He offers treatments to his current patient base, adds a section about dental implants to his website, and invests
in a logo, signage, and print ads. He even develops a micro-website on the
topic. Basically, he made the same marketing choices as his colleague near
Houston. Would he be successful?

Let's look at the demographics of these dentists' areas, in contrast to their
ideal patient or target market.

Suburban Houston

Community Demographics	Target Market Demographics
50% female	Male or female
30% male	Primarily age 50+
20% kids	Primarily white
Young families	$80K+/household
White/Hispanic	Mostly white collar
$60K/year, one income	Insurance, CareCredit,
75% blue collar	or credit card
25%white collar	
30% insured	
70% uninsured	

Metro Seattle

Community Demographics	Target Market Demographics
35% female	Male or female
65% male	Primarily age 50+
Executives age 30–70	Primarily white
White/Hispanic	$80K+/household
$120K/year	Mostly white collar
98% white collar	Insurance, CareCredit,
70% insured	or credit card
30% uninsured	

According to the information in these charts, the Seattle dentist may have more success with a niche practice focusing on dental implants. The Houston dentist should consider alternatives. With his community demographics, perhaps clear braces for teens and adults or fast braces would be more successful.

Smart Business Tip—*Understanding what a patient needs and the associated psychology of case acceptance will be crucial in properly executing your niche. A new book on the market, THE ART OF CASE PRESENTATION by Barry F. Polansky, DMD (2013), is an excellent source of up-to-date information on this topic.*

What You Need to Know to Make the Right Choice

How can you know which niche would meet the needs and achieve the goals of your community's members? What do you need to know to make a wise choice regarding the niche practice you should invest in? In the following sections, we'll discuss the target market demographics for some of the most successful and profitable niches in dentistry. We'll also provide guidelines you can use to do your own market research.

Actions to Take

- Consider which niches interest you.
- Analyze your community demographics.
- Think about which of the niches that interest you might yield the most profit per hour of chair time.
- Search the Internet to determine if your colleagues offer those treatments in your community.
- Conduct pricing research by calling your competitors.
- Test your choice of niches with a trial run.

Smart Business Tip— *Test your market by offering limited-scope niche services and gauging demand. No matter what outside research tells you, it is wise to fire some "test bullets" before you fire cannonballs in developing the niche.*

Special Services to Consider

This guide includes the following special services:

- Cosmetic Dentistry
- Dental Implants
- Mini Dental Implants
- Orthodontics
- Endodontics and Extractions
- CEREC Same-Day Crowns
- Laser Dentistry

Cosmetic Dentistry

Cosmetic dental services—

Cosmetic dentistry can refer to purely cosmetic services, like veneers and whitening, but more often, the term is used to describe any dental procedure that enhances appearance. We might say that cosmetic dentures, cosmetic crowns (ceramic or zirconia), or cosmetic fillings (composites) are examples of such procedures. A *smile makeover* describes any treatment plan that includes dental procedures to improve the overall appearance of a smile. Given this, bridges, gum lifts, and bonding fall under the umbrella of cosmetic dentistry.

General demographics of the cosmetic dental patient—

According to the American Academy of Cosmetic Dentistry's publication, *Cosmetic Dentistry State of the Industry Survey 2011*, esthetic dental procedures are no longer just for women. The survey of seven hundred to nine hundred dentists (depending on the question) showed that men make up 40 percent of all cosmetic dental patients in the United States. The average age of most patients ranges from thirty-one to sixty, though the number of cosmetic dental patients under twenty is on the rise.

The aging baby boomers and their inherent desire for youthful appearance will drive up the demand for cosmetic dental services over the next decade. Services likes teeth whitening, dentures, and implants will see brisk demand from the "forever young at heart" crowd. Aligning your practice to serve this all-important aging demographic will be crucial, especially if your office is located in an area where many seniors retire.

In fact, whitening is the most requested dental procedure in America today. The American Dental Association (ADA) estimates that over one billion dollars are spent annually on professional whitening treatments.

What's important to the patient—

Continuing with the American Academy of Dentistry (AACD) 2011 survey findings, the most important factors to cosmetic dental patients are:

- Their appearance
- Cost of the procedures
- Longevity of the treatment
- Potential for pain
- Time required for treatment
- Amount of natural tooth structure that has to be reduced prior to a procedure

What patients spend on cosmetic dentistry—

Here's good news if you're considering a niche practice in cosmetic dentistry. Doctors who saw cosmetic patients report that 25 percent spent more than $2,500 in a single visit. Per year, 19 percent of cosmetic patients spent between $2,500 and $5,000. Over two-thirds of the dentists who responded to the 2011 AACD survey reported offering third-party financing, such as CareCredit or Chase Health Advance. As for total profits, the survey says that about a quarter of dentists report earning between $100,000 and $249,000 annually from cosmetic procedures, another quarter earned between $250,000 and $499,000, and just under a quarter earned less than $100,000. Who made over a million? Survey says, 6 percent.

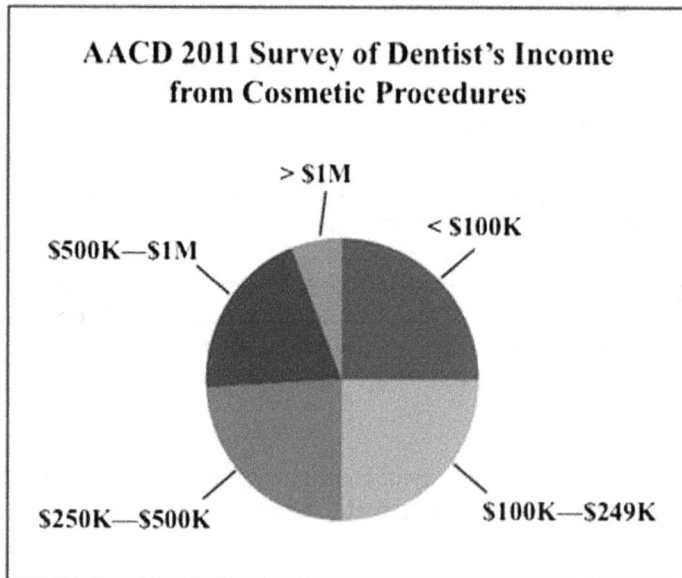

AACD 2011 Survey of Dentist's Income from Cosmetic Procedures

> $1M
$500K—$1M
< $100K
$250K—$500K
$100K—$249K

Dental Implants

Dental implant services—

From a patient's perspective, dental implants are an invasive, two-part procedure that involves the placement of an implant post and then securing a prosthetic, separated by a healing phase. Dentists who place *or* restore implants can call themselves implant dentists because the American Dental Association does not require specialty designation. All prosthodontists, periodontists, and oral surgeons can place implant posts, though general dentists can become trained to perform implant placement surgery.

General demographics of the dental implant patient—

In 2006, *Dental Economics* published that thirty million Americans have no teeth. According to the American Academy of Implant Dentistry (AAID), 69 percent of patients age thirty-five to forty-four have lost one or more teeth, and by age seventy-four, over one-quarter are edentulous. Experts predict that the population of Americans over age fifty-five will nearly double by 2030, going from 20 percent to 30 percent of the entire population. To the implant dentist, this means a growing customer base.

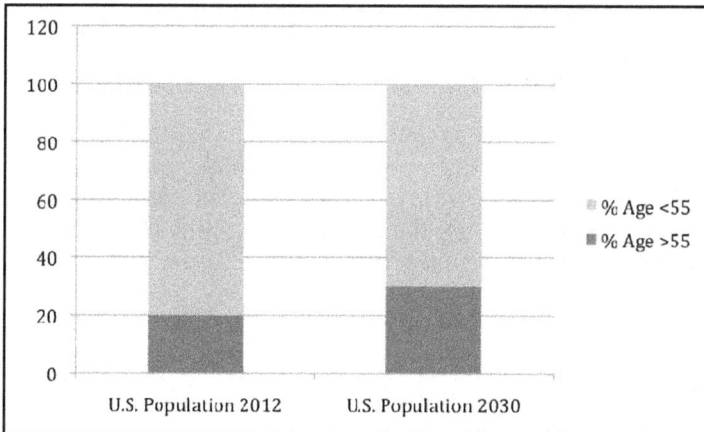

The AAID also tells us that three million people have dental implants, and half a million are added to this number annually. Because dental implants can replace a single tooth or anchor a bridge, partial, or denture, they can meet the needs of patients with any number of missing teeth.

In corporate America, when such powerful demographic research becomes available, competitive companies adapt and start developing long-term strategies for entering and succeeding in a new market. Why can't a dentist borrow a page from the corporate playbook and take the logical next step?

The ability to offer implants enhances the personal brand value of the general dentist. It allows you to distance yourself from many individual dentists and large group practices who offer dentistry as a commodity rather than a lifestyle enhancement experience.

What's important to the patient—

In the 1960s, people lived an average of sixty-five years, but today we live nearly two decades longer. In fact, over sixty-six thousand Americans are centenarians—meaning that they are more than one hundred years old. Quality of life, the ability to consume a healthy diet, and self-confidence depend in part on proper oral function and appearance. Some research even suggests that edentulous people do not live as long as those with a full set of healthy teeth.

Dentures are one option for replacing all teeth, but studies show that dentures are not ideal. In fact, many denture patients do not wear both of their dentures, and some don't wear their dentures at all. Common causes cited for dislike and noncompliance are slippage, discomfort, the inconvenience of removing and cleaning them, and the cost of refitting and replacing them.

To replace a single tooth, a bridge or partial has long been the standard. However, both of these prosthetics rely on healthy teeth for support. For bridge placement, healthy tooth structure must be altered for crown placement. Bridges and partials compromise the integrity of healthy teeth and can contribute to further tooth loss or dental problems in the future.

In contrast to dentures, partials, and bridges, dental implants imitate nature's design. With a prosthetic root and crown, a successful dental implant does not slip or loosen over time. It performs better with biting forces and, with proper care, can last a lifetime.

A February 2013 Global Business Intelligence report, titled "Technological Advancements and Elderly Populations Lead to Increased Preference for Dental Implants," indicated that the US dental implant market would be slightly under $1 billion in 2013. Based on demographic trends and technological advances, GBI Research projected that the dental implant market will double by 2018 to almost $2 billion. These trends, coupled with the fact that more general practitioners are placing implants, cannot be ignored.

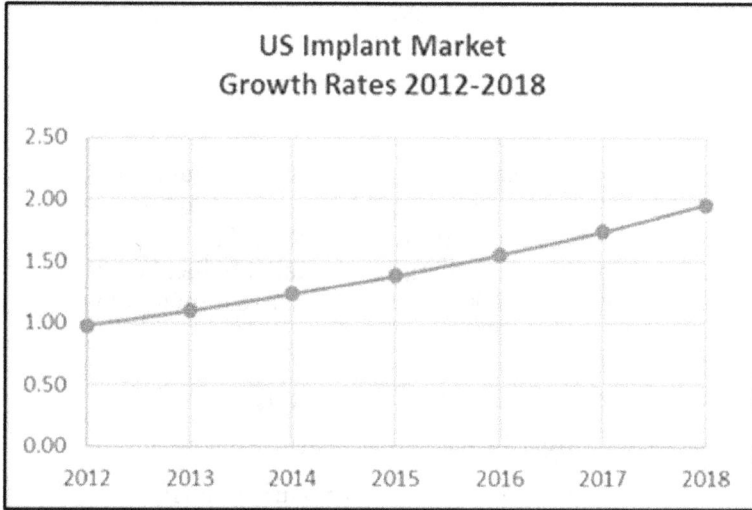

US Implant Market Growth Rates 2012-2018

	2012	2013	2014	2015	2016	2017	2018

What patients spend on dental implants—

A 2010 article by Lesley Alderman in the New York Times, "For Most, Implants Beat Dentures, but at a Price," *reported that a single tooth replacement by dental implant costs $3,000 to $4,500, and replacing multiple or all teeth can cost between $20,000 and $45,000. An article at* http://health. costhelper.com/dental-implant.html *reveals that implant patients pay up to $80,000 for full upper and lower dentures. Health and dental insurance do not cover the full cost of dental implants, so implant dentists are wise to offer patient financing.*

Mini Dental Implants

Recently approved by the FDA, mini dental implants (MDIs) can be used as both transitional and long-term devices for stabilizing a dental prosthesis. At less than 3 millimeters in diameter, mini implants can even be appropriate for patients whose compromised jawbone density excludes them from qualifying for conventional dental implant placement. Training courses for MDIs generally only require a weekend or two. Furthermore, your initial investment in materials and a kit is reasonable given the potential return on investment MDIs can generate. To illustrate the potential boon a mini implant niche could prove for your practice, consider the following scenarios:

• **Scenario 1:** Your patient comes into the office with a severely fractured tooth that's causing some discomfort and seriously impeding his or her ability to carry on normally. You perform an extraction and a bone graft, place the mini implant and abutment, and bond a temporary crown. Your patient walks out of the building with a functional, realistic new tooth, and you've successfully made nearly $4,000 for an approximately two-hour procedure.

• **Scenario 2:** Your patient schedules a consultation because a loose bottom denture continues to embarrass her in social situations. You place a mini dental implant to stabilize the denture. She leaves the office with renewed confidence and improved quality of life. You've just earned between $850 and $1,000 for about forty-five minutes of your time.

Sleep Apnea and Snoring Cessation Treatments

Dental sleep medicine services—

For many years, continuous positive airway pressure (CPAP) has been the standard treatment for sleep apnea. If CPAP did not prove effective for the patient, surgery may have been recommended. Both of these treatments remain prevalent today, but dental sleep medicine has also entered the arena.

While snoring is not a sure indicator of sleep apnea, it is definitely a symptom. Many people who snore have sleep apnea, and the most common type of sleep apnea is obstructive sleep apnea, or OSA. Dentists who offer sleep apnea and snoring treatment cannot diagnose sleep apnea. However, they can provide a patient with a referral to a sleep lab or a home sleep study kit.

Sleep medicine doctors, including dentists, offer an oral appliance that holds the lower jaw slightly forward to keep the airway clear during sleep. This slight anatomical adjustment often alleviates snoring and OSA symptoms.

General demographics of the sleep apnea or snoring patient—

While studies are not consistent, experts believe that 30 to 50 percent of the population snores, and snoring becomes more prevalent as one's age and weight increase. Sleep apnea affects approximately eighteen million people in the United States, and men are more likely to suffer from obstructive sleep apnea than women.

What's important to the patient—

Snoring in and of itself can interrupt sleep for both the snorer and his or her sleeping partner. Studies show serious quality-of-life issues for snorers and their bedmates. These include, but are not limited to, hearing problems, sleep deprivation, irritability, and poor daytime productivity. According to research by the Mayo Clinic, after treatment for snoring, the snorer and the bedmate can experience improved quality of life within six weeks.

For patients who also suffer with OSA, health problems can include increased risk for high blood pressure, cardiovascular disease, premature death, cognitive problems, weight gain, headaches or migraines, difficulty concentrating, falling asleep at times of low stimulation, and impotence. For some occupations, such as driving, sleep apnea can alter a person's ability to perform job duties.

Recent evidence has demonstrated a clear link between oral health and overall health. Creating a holistic approach to patient health will enhance your reputation among your patients and the local community—thereby enhancing your standing as a highly qualified expert.

What patients spend on snoring and sleep apnea treatment—

Diagnosis requires a home sleep study or overnight stay at a sleep lab. The home kit generally costs $200 to $300 (with a co-pay of $30). A night in a sleep lab can run $2,000 (with a co-pay of $320 to $1,000). A CPAP machine costs $150 to $5,000 or more, though a monthly co-pay on rental may run only $120. Maintenance, which involves replacing the mask and tubing on a CPAP unit, generally costs $200 every six months. The oral appliances prescribed by dental sleep medicine practitioners range from $700 to $2,500 and may also include an annual maintenance visit and charge. In some cases, health insurance covers some of the cost of sleep apnea diagnosis and treatment, as well as oral appliances.

Overall, sleep disorder diagnoses and treatments are on the rise. We see this trend in Medicare payments for sleep disorders, which increased from $62 million in 2001 to $235 million in 2009. In 2011, Americans doled out $1.7 billion on prescription sleep drugs. According to IBISWorld, Inc., the sleep medicine market will grow 9 percent annually, reaching $9 billion by 2018.

Smart Business Tip—*Diagnosis and basic treatment, including the oral appliance, take very little of your time and produce an additional revenue stream per chair hour.*

Orthodontics

Orthodontic services provided by nonorthodontists—

While general dentists and orthodontists debate over who can better serve a patient in need of orthodontic treatment, all general dentists receive training in orthodontics during their regular course of study in dental school and in most cases, can confidently place traditional braces.

With recent advances in accelerated orthodontic treatments, more general and family dentists have expanded their practices to include systems such as:

- Invisalign
- ClearCorrect
- Six Month Smiles
- Cfast

These systems require some formal training, usually completed in the course of a weekend or daylong seminar, and allow dentists to treat mild-to-moderate spacing and alignment issues for most patients. More importantly, these systems generally require six months to one year to complete treatment as opposed to the eighteen months to three years required for traditional braces.

General demographics of nonspecialist orthodontics—

Patients seek orthodontic treatment to improve both their overall oral health and the appearance of their teeth. About four million Americans currently wear some variety of orthodontics and approximately one million of those wearers are adults over the age of eighteen.

While we tend to associate braces and orthodontics with children and teens, a growing number of image-conscious adults are seeking orthodontic treatment to straighten their teeth and enhance the esthetic of their smiles. It stands to reason that these patients will seek out clear or nearly invisible orthodontic options, since walking around with a "metal mouth" for eighteen months to three years won't appeal to most adults active on the professional and social scene.

What's important to the patient—

For the most part, adults seek orthodontic treatment for cosmetic reasons. Put plainly, crooked and uneven teeth aren't appealing and can make people appear to be in poor health or older than their age. Many of these patients may have needed orthodontics as children or teens but were unable to undergo treatment due to family resources or other reasons.

As the job market remains sluggish, seasoned professionals and first-time job seekers understand the impact a nice smile can have on their marketability. Furthermore, improving the appearance of one's smile can significantly impact the quality of interpersonal and romantic interactions. According to a survey conducted by the Max Planck Institute in Berlin and reported in the journal *Psychology and Aging* (June 2012), straight teeth and a genuine smile make a person look younger.

Many accelerated orthodontic systems, such as Invisalign, ClearCorrect, and Six Month Smiles offer clear or nearly invisible treatment. Offering these treatment options gives you a clear advantage over dentists and orthodontists who offer only unsightly, traditional metal braces.

Most patients will also appreciate the reduced treatment time required of most of these systems. For instance, Invisalign can correct most spacing and alignment problems in about a year, if the patient closely follows your treatment plan. Six Month Smiles can correct cosmetic issues in the front teeth in as little as, wait for it, six months.

What patients spend on fast, removable, cosmetic braces—

Traditional metal braces cost an average of $3,000 to $6,000, depending on region and each patient's specific needs. Clear Invisalign aligners cost an average of $5,000 and offer the added benefits of removability, ease of cleaning, and improved esthetics. ClearCorrect, another brand of clear plastic aligners, offers the same benefits and general cost as Invisalign. Six Month Smiles, a new type of affixed braces that utilize clear brackets and white wires, can cost anywhere between $2,000 and $4,000, depending on the needs of the patient. The resulting profit margins are among the best of any healthcare procedure.

> *Smart Business Tip*—*From a case acceptance perspective, orthodontics is the easiest for patients to accept, especially when it's for their children. If you do a great job for the children, parents will follow suit.*

Endodontics and Extractions

Endodontic therapy and extractions—

Endodontics, more commonly referred to as *root canals* or *root canal therapy*, provides a restorative option for patients suffering from advanced tooth decay or severe trauma that has put the tooth pulp in jeopardy. Endodontic therapy provides immediate relief from the pain associated with exposed pulp and saves the structure of the tooth not affected by damage or decay. Extraction procedures can vary in complexity and may be necessary for several reasons, including trauma, advanced gum disease, severe tooth decay beyond the power of endodontic therapy, preparation for orthodontic treatment, and reducing the risk of infection in patients with impaired immune function.

General demographics of the endodontic and extraction patient—

According to the American Association of Endodontists, general dentists and specialists perform approximately fourteen million root canal procedures per year in the United States and enjoy a 95 percent success rate. The majority of endodontic procedures are performed on adult patients, although children with severe decay or tooth trauma may qualify.

Although we cannot know the true number, dental health experts estimate that dentists extract nearly twenty million teeth in the United States every year. Since people across the age spectrum may need a tooth pulled, extractions truly fit the family dentist's scope of care.

What's important to the patient—

Root canal therapy suffers from the undeserved reputation for being painful. Most patients will feel nervous or afraid when you recommend this procedure, so you will want to focus on alleviating their anxiety. Root canal therapy is performed under local anesthesia and, once completed, will actually alleviate the discomfort and pain associated with exposed pulp tissue. Helping patients understand the restorative nature of this procedure and its ability to save the tooth's structure may reduce some anxiety.

Similarly, patient concerns about tooth extractions will focus primarily on the level of discomfort they can expect and how long the healing process will require. Patients can expect to have the extraction site fully numbed and can ask their dentist about sedative options. After an extraction, complete healing will generally require several weeks to a few months, although the site will feel comfortable enough to return to normal function within a few days. How closely a patient follows postoperative instructions for caring for the extraction site will determine the success and rapidity of healing.

You may also want to take the opportunity to discuss tooth replacement options with your patient. Implant-supported crowns and bridges will restore the function, health, and appearance of your patient's smile.

What patients spend on endodontic therapy and extractions—

Endodontic therapy can range anywhere from $300 to $2,000 per tooth, depending on the severity of the case and the tooth's placement in the dental arch. Extractions can vary from as little as $100 to as high as $900 per tooth, depending on whether a simple or surgical extraction is required.

> **Smart Business Tip**—Combining a root canal with a restorative crown can significantly enhance your revenue while reducing the cost of another appointment, another anesthetic, and extra front office time.

CEREC Same-Day Crowns

A dental crown provides support and restores the structure of a compromised tooth. Perfect for treating cracked or damaged teeth, or a tooth that has undergone root canal therapy, crowns can also serve as a beautiful, highly realistic cosmetic solution for patients who do not qualify for veneers.

CEREC CAD/CAM technology—

CEREC technology from Sirona utilizes computer-assisted design and manufacturing to create all-porcelain crowns that you can place in a single visit. After preparing the tooth enamel, you take digital impressions of the tooth and surrounding structure to upload to the computer. Using its software, you design a custom-fitted crown. You send the design from the computer to a special milling machine that creates the crown from a block of dental ceramic or resin. At present, there are five types of blocks used for CEREC restorations: feldspathic porcelain, leucite porcelain, lithium disilicate, resin composite, and zirconium oxide. The composite materials are often used for temporary prosthetics. After milling, you can stain, glaze, and fire the crown to enhance its strength and esthetics before placing.

Some traditionalists question whether CEREC crowns, milled from single blocks of porcelain, can offer the same natural translucence of a layered, lab-created crown. In answer to these concerns, most dentists opt to stain and glaze their CEREC crowns to color-match and enhance the reflectivity of the porcelain. When handled by a dentist with an artistic eye, CEREC crowns look indistinguishable from lab-made crowns. As many CEREC dentists point out, they can achieve a better color-matched restoration with the patient sitting in the chair, rather than by sending a picture to the lab.

General demographics of the CEREC same-day crown patient—

According to the American College of Prosthodontics, approximately 178 million American adults have lost at least one tooth to gum disease, tooth decay, extractions, or accidental injury. Experts estimate that number will increase to two hundred million over the next fifteen years as the population ages. Many of these partially edentulous people will seek out tooth replacement options to restore the look and function of their mouths, and dentists who provide CEREC same-day crowns are poised to provide treatment for these patients.

What's important to the patient—

Most patients will look forward to the dramatically reduced wait time and increased convenience involved in placing CEREC crowns. Traditional crowns require at least two separate visits to the office. Additionally, the patient has to wear a temporary crown while waiting for the permanent crown to arrive from the lab. If the temporary crown should fail before the permanent one arrives, the patient will need to make time for another appointment. Avoiding the use of ill-fitting and often faulty temporary crowns will enhance a patient's overall experience. If, however, a provisional crown is indicated for a trial period, one can be CEREC-milled from resin composite.

What patients spend on CEREC same-day crown treatment—

Patients can expect to spend an average of $1,000 per crown. Of course, that fee will vary depending on the material used, as well as staining and glazing the crown for enhanced strength and esthetics.

> *Smart Business Tip—CEREC is a great marketing tool as it enhances patient perception of your practice as a high-quality and state-of-the-art. If you choose to offer it, feature it prominently in your marketing.*

Laser Dentistry

Laser dental procedures—

Comprised of a concentrated beam of light energy, dental lasers allow dentists to safely and accurately treat a number of hard- and soft-tissue concerns. Some common uses for dental lasers include:

- Removing inflamed or infected gingival tissue in the treatment of gum disease
- Reshaping the gum line to improve the overall smile esthetics and assist in placing porcelain veneers
- Alleviating the discomfort associated with cold or canker sores
- Treating bacterial infections within the pulp
- Activating teeth-whitening treatments

Dental lasers allow you to avoid the use of anesthetic in some cases, reduce healing time and bleeding, and provide more precise treatment.

General demographics of the laser dentistry patient—

Since clinical applications of laser dentistry fall into different categories of dental care, determining the demographics of the laser dentistry patient presents something of a challenge. However, a good deal of laser therapy will focus on treating gum disease, and 50 percent of Americans over the age of thirty suffer from this disorder. The average general or family dentist is apt to see several cases per day in which a dental laser can provide an appropriate solution.

What's important to the patient—

The foremost concern among patients facing dental laser therapy is pain. They assume laser treatment will hurt. In reality, dental lasers often remove the need for local anesthetic, and because lasers seal the soft tissues as they move along the gums, patients experience little or no bleeding. As opposed to traditional techniques that require cutting and stitching, laser gum treatments offer a far more gentle option and greatly reduce discomfort, swelling, and healing time. Lasers also allow for more precise treatments. For example, performing a gum lift using traditional tools does not allow for the enhanced precision offered by soft-tissue lasers. Using a laser, a dentist can preserve more of the natural tissue, thus providing a more conservative treatment option.

What patients spend on laser dentistry treatment—

The cost of dental laser treatments will vary from procedure to procedure. However, the average cost of a laser gum lift can vary from $75 to $175 per tooth. Periodontal disease therapy using a laser can run up to $6,000 for a full-mouth case but, when compared to the cost of replacing a tooth or several teeth lost to gum disease, the price of therapy seems well worth it.

Your Community Demographics

You need to establish a solid understanding of your community, its people, and your current patient base so that you can apply demographic data to your marketing strategy. Knowledge is power, and knowing your potential and current patients will enable you to make informed marketing decisions for your practice.

Here are the items you will need to research:

1. Which towns, regions, and zip codes are within twelve to twenty miles of your dental practice?

2. For each of these towns or regions, note the following data (use www.city-data.com or a similar free tool to acquire the information):

- Population
- Median age
- Percent female, male, and children
- Percent of married and unmarried people
- Number in household
- Median income
- Percent of renters versus homeowners
- Home value
- Percent of single family versus multifamily residences
- Population percentages by race

3. Which companies are the largest employers? Do you accept their insurance? Are you in network?

4. What are the largest entertainment facilities in your area?

5. What are the most popular clubs, associations, or organizations in your area? (Schools, sports, religious institutions, women's groups, country clubs, etc.)

6. Look at your current patient data. In which cities, regions, or zip codes do most of your patients live?

7. What is the breakdown, by percentage, of males, females, and children?

8. What is the median age of your current patient base?

9. Are most of your patients single or married?

10. What is the median income level of your current patient base? (You may have to guess.)

11. What percentage of your patients pay by each of the following: cash or check, credit card, financing, and insurance?

12. What were the most popular procedures that your office performed last year?

13. What were the most profitable procedures that your office performed last year?

14. What amount of fees did you have to write off last year, and which procedures were they for?

Now you have a good understanding of your community members and current patients, what their lives entail, what they value, and what they will invest in. Compare this information with the niche practices you're considering, and determine which niche might best serve the needs and meet the goals of your community members and current patients.

Next Steps

1. Define your community demographics.

2. Define your current patient demographics.

3. Decide which niches interest you.

4. Compare the demographics of your selected niches to those of your community and current patients.

5. Decide which niches will best serve your community, patients, and practice.

Chapter Two:
Preparing for Success

Success in business requires training and discipline and hard work.
But, if these things do not frighten you, the opportunities are just as
great today as they ever were.
—David Rockefeller

Training and Equipment

Your initial and ongoing investment in the equipment, materials, and training necessary to expand your niche practice will vary depending on which
services you want to provide. Having a firm understanding of the total cost
of your investment, as well as a realistic idea of your target demographic
based on the market research you performed, will allow you to make an informed decision. Financially speaking, your most straightforward goal is to
invest in the niche that will provide you with the best return-on-investment
(ROI). Expressed as a percentage, you can calculate ROI with the following
equation:

ROI = (Gain from Investment–Cost of Investment)/
Cost of Investment

Of course, at this stage, your equation and ROI are well-informed estimates
that may not include other benefits, such as the increased productivity of
your hygiene staff or improved overall marketability of your practice. The
following offers a general overview of the basic equipment, training, materials, and related purchases you will need to make. As you move closer to making a decision on your niche practice, we encourage you to research further.

Cosmetic Dentistry

First, you will need to consider which cosmetic treatments you want to offer.
Most dental practices with a minimal cosmetic menu provide veneers, teeth
whitening or bleaching systems, and cosmetic dental bonding.

• *Veneers*—Consider which types of veneers you would like to offer. Choices include resin veneers, traditional porcelain veneers, and no-prep or minimal-prep ultra-thin veneers. Do you want to partner with a well-known brand, such as daVinci or Lumineers, which offers built-in name recognition? Or would you prefer to work with a smaller, private ceramist? In addition to the costs associated with partnering with a ceramist, you will have to purchase enamel preparation tools, impression materials, and cementing and bonding materials.

Training—As with many dental procedures, cosmetic and otherwise, you will need to take a dynamic approach to veneers training, one that includes weekend courses and seminars, over-the-shoulder training, model work, and live patient training. As you become more familiar and adept at veneer placement, consider advanced training to further hone your skills.

• *Teeth whitening*—First, you will need to decide whether you want to offer take-home whitening trays, in-office whitening, or a combination of both. Materials associated with take-home whitening trays include tray materials, model kits, vacuum-forming machines, and a selection of prefilled syringes in a variety of gel strengths. Materials associated with in-office whitening include whitening gels, syringes, disposable tips, desensitizing gels, gingival dams, shade charts, and curing lights.

Training—In addition to offering a relatively low-cost investment, most teeth-whitening systems require minimal training. Branded systems may require that you and your staff attend a seminar or training course but, for the most part, whitening procedures require the same basic steps.

• *Cosmetic bonding*—Like whitening systems, cosmetic bonding can be added to your services menu at a relatively low cost. No doubt you have already invested in the needed shaping and polishing burs and a quality handset. Your most important decision will involve choosing which brand or variety of composite resin you want to work with. You have hundreds of options, and you should choose the one that offers the best durability, workability, and esthetics at the best cost for you. Furthermore, many companies offer BPA-free resins that may appeal to your health and environmentally conscious target demographic.

Training—Since you probably already know the basics of using composite resin, your training may involve more case identification training than hands-on application. Knowing when bonding is appropriate and when to recommend other treatments reasserts your professional authority and instills confidence in your patients.

Dental Implants

With the right demographic and marketing tools in place, a dental implant niche can have a huge impact on your practice's bottom line. Expanding your practice to include dental implants depends on having a clear plan for what you want to provide. Specifically, do you want to restore implants or do you hope to one day perform all aspects of dental implantation, from planning through surgery and restoration? Most general dentists begin their dental implant practice by partnering with a trusted oral surgeon for implant and abutment placement. In addition, you will need to partner with a talented ceramist and prosthodontics studio so you can provide the types of restorations you and your patients want.

Training—After finishing dental school, you have the training necessary to restore dental implants. However, only experience and further training can prepare you for complications or issues that may arise during the restoration process. As you gain more experience and acquire a better understanding of exactly how profitable dental implants can be for your practice, you may decide to receive more advanced training in dental implants. Comprehensive training or fellowship programs are offered throughout the United States to help general dentists expand their experience and knowledge in dental implantology.

Sleep Apnea and Snoring Cessation Treatment

Several aspects of a sleep apnea or snoring treatment niche that you will need to consider include:

- Partnering with a nearby sleep lab to which to refer patients who need sleep tests.
- Offering take-home sleep apnea tests that will help patients avoid the need for overnight stays at a sleep lab.
- The types of sleep apnea and snoring devices you choose to offer and which manufacturer you will trust to provide these devices. These can include mandibular advancement devices or tongue retraining devices. Spending the time to conduct some research in this area can mean the difference between a successful sleep apnea and snoring niche and an underperforming one.

Training—For the most part, training for the treatment of sleep apnea and snoring will require learning the basics of fitting devices and case identification. You will need to refer most severe cases of sleep apnea to medical specialists. Furthermore, if you choose to offer lifestyle modification advice as part of a comprehensive sleep apnea treatment plan, you will need adequate information about diet and exercise changes your patients can make.

Orthodontics

First, you will need to decide which types and brands of accelerated orthodontic treatment would best serve the needs of your practice and your patients. Your two most common options include clear aligners, such as Invisalign and ClearCorrect, and fixed cosmetic braces, such as Six Month Smiles and Cfast. Many general dentists offer one brand of each type of accelerated orthodontics in order to reach out to a wider candidate group.

Training—Each brand will offer training seminars for different experience levels, as well as online resources for dentists and patients. One of the greatest challenges facing general dentists new to accelerated orthodontics, or orthodontics of any kind, is proper case identification. Successfully determining which patients qualify for accelerated treatment and which patients require the services of an orthodontist will help you better serve your patients and create a positive buzz about your services.

Endodontics and Extractions

If you choose to expand your practice to include root canal therapy or extractions, you will first need to determine the level of care you want to provide. Most general dentists perform straightforward root canal therapy and simple extractions. Developing your endodontic practice may include gaining more experience in and becoming more comfortable with performing root canal therapy on patients with more complex root structures.

Growing an extraction niche may include gaining experience and training on the extractions of wisdom teeth and impacted teeth, tooth sectioning, and surgical extractions. You may not need to make any major investments in equipment outside of different types of forceps. However, you may need to alter your sedation and anesthetic program to accommodate more complex procedures.

Training—Mastering more complex endodontic procedures and extractions requires a blended approach, one that includes hands-on courses, over-the-shoulder training, model work, and live patient training. Professional organizations such as the Academy of General Dentistry can offer training opportunities, as can an endodontist in your area.

CEREC Same-Day Crowns

Opening a same-day crown niche within your general dentistry practice represents both a big investment and a big opportunity for practice growth. A CEREC system costs approximately $100,000, and, with an average five-year lease, you can expect to pay about $2,000 per month for the equipment. Additional supplies include design and workflow software, hardware and software for taking digital impressions, milling burs, dental porcelain blocks, stains, and glazes. In addition, you will need to schedule regular maintenance and upgrades for the equipment and software.

Training—The best technology in the world is useless without a properly trained person to operate it. CEREC training offers hands-on education at every level of experience. Courses you and your staff can expect to attend include orientation, basic through advanced techniques, integration with other systems, CEREC-specific marketing strategies, and solutions for successfully integrating CEREC into your practice.

Smart Business Tip—*Understanding current tax laws can significantly benefit your equipment purchase decisions. Accelerated depreciation deductions can dramatically reduce the economic cost of a purchase. Consulting your dental CPA is a must for making smart, tax-friendly decisions.*

Laser Dentistry

Laser dentistry can enhance the accuracy and precision of patient care that your practice provides, and your initial investment will depend on the treatments you wish to offer. If you only plan on performing soft-tissue treatments such as gum contouring or periodontal disease treatments, you will need to purchase a dental diode laser system. Dental diodes generally run between $2,000 and $5,000 and can be purchased used or new through a variety of reputable online dealers. If you want to make laser dentistry a prominent part of your practice, you may want to consider investing in a laser that can perform soft- and hard-tissue procedures, such as the Waterlase MD Turbo by Biolase. While these more complex laser systems may cost upward of $17,000, you can expect to incorporate this system into several areas of your practice.

Training—The Academy of Laser Dentistry (ALD) offers a comprehensive selection of online courses, certifications, and training seminars for dentists interested in expanding their knowledge and technique. Before investing in your dental laser, consider taking an orientation and standard proficiency course with the ALD to make sure that you have a firm grasp of the basics. This will allow you to make a more informed decision before investing.

Becoming the Expert

You've bought the equipment, stocked the materials, and you and your team have received the basic training needed to start offering your newest services. So how do you make the transition from a dentist who merely offers a niche service to a dentist recognized as a local expert for that service?

The Internet and related technologies, including chat, social media, and net-meetings, have enabled today's consumer to reach a completely different level of sophistication. Consumers have practically any kind of information literally at their fingertips.

Businesses and individuals who have achieved success within the professional-services world have leveraged the power of technology to enhance their brand or reputation to earn substantially higher profits. Establishing a personal brand is a necessity in today's highly competitive world where sophisticated consumers are inundated by a slew of highly customized information delivered directly to their desktops, laptops, tablets, and mobile phones.

Establishing a personal brand is a two-step process. First, it requires an investment in time and a commitment to professional improvement, that is, obtaining the necessary know-how to become a true technical expert in your field of expertise. Second, it involves engaging in effective self-promotion that creates a perception among the community and your patients that you are the superior dentist in your area.

Advanced Training Experience

Luckily, you have an endless assortment of seminars, classes, and training sessions offered by clinics, universities, and brand representatives to choose from. Make the most of these readily available resources by dedicating a part of your yearly budget to professional development for you and your team. To get the most benefit from your trainings, follow these guidelines:

- Don't forget to take a dynamic approach to your training. Incorporate over-the-shoulder training and model work with lectures and hands-on training.
- Identify experts and established dentists whose work you want to emulate and attend their workshops.
- Don't forget to brush up on business and marketing for your niche. After all, part of becoming an expert means letting people know about your expertise.

Professional Association Fellowships

Patients interpret your membership in a professional organization as a sign of your dedication to professional development. Many professional associations offer fellowship programs that encourage dentists to push their clinical skills to a higher level. To earn a fellowship, members generally have to demonstrate association membership, perform a certain number of cases, earn extra continuing education hours, present patient before-and-after photos, and complete an examination. Not only does receiving a fellowship help you hone your skills and give you a well-earned sense of accomplishment, it lets your patients know that you have been recognized for your dedication and skill.

Develop a Local Referral Network

Referral networks help you establish a mutually beneficial relationship with another professional and can help you grow both your patient base and your reputation as an expert. Establishing that network will require some footwork both in your community and in an online environment.

Take advantage of community events and the local or regional chapters of national dental associations, as well as online message and discussion boards.

Training the Team

Leadership is the art of getting someone else to do something you want done because he wants to do it.
—*Dwight Eisenhower*

Getting Staff Buy-In

Taking your dental practice in a new direction will prove a source of excitement for most of your team. Just the prospect of getting to open up a new piece of equipment or learn a new procedure can lend the office an air of anticipation and fun. Other employees may feel reserved, doubtful, intimidated, or downright hostile to the changes that come as you transition your practice. Getting your team on board is essential to the successful deployment of your new services. The following steps can help you move the entire staff toward buy-in:

1. Present your case at a staff meeting. With all team members present, discuss your plan for expanding the practice, how these changes will help everyone provide better patient care, and how this new or enhanced service corresponds to your practice's guiding mission or philosophy.

2. Foster enthusiasm and confidence by presenting a well-thought-out plan. Discuss with your team how you intend to implement these new changes in clear steps. You may also want to present a timeline for implementation.

3. Invite feedback. During the meeting, ask for questions, comments, or even gut reactions. Encourage your staff to talk or e-mail you if any concerns or questions should arise. Help your employees feel involved and personally invested in seeing their workplace develop and improve.

Educating the Educators

Your hygienists, assistants, and office coordinators provide frontline marketing for your new niche services. They enjoy more face-to-face time with patients and therefore have a better opportunity to educate patients on the full range of services you can provide. Ensuring that your staff receives adequate training in the benefits, costs, and treatment details can result in the enhanced visibility and profitability of your niche.

> *Smart Business Tip*—*An annual training retreat that includes classroom training as well as team-building exercises can be an effective strategy to instill confidence in your staff and give them the necessary tools to enhance customer experience and thereby increase your bottom line.*

The value of education for patients and staff—

In terms of general results, patient education helps people enjoy better health and an enhanced quality of life. Specifically, patient education can secure better clinical outcomes and better at-home care. In addition, educated patients feel more invested in the dentist–patient relationship, are far more likely to seek out regular preventive care, and look to treatment for outstanding issues.

Look at it this way: patient education provides a significant source of professional satisfaction for your hygienists, assistants, and front office staff who think of developing trusting patient relationships as one of the most important features of their jobs. **Very often, dental staff members are unfamiliar with the importance and requirements of communicating effectively.** In addition, patients are often turned off by staff members who can't effectively answer their questions. Patient education provides a valuable sales solution that also fulfills your staff members' dedication to patient care.

Patient education as a marketing tool—

How can patient education provide an effective marketing tool for your new niche service? Here are the top three ways:

- First, patient education offers a relatively inexpensive marketing solution since it takes place during the normal course of an appointment and does not require any special materials, although additional resources such as brochures or imaging software may prove helpful once your niche takes off.
- Second, one-on-one patient education is personalized marketing. When you and your staff recommend services based on your patients' unique needs, it reinforces a solid patient relationship. When your

patients trust you, they are more likely to follow your advice regarding care and treatment.
- Third, patient education is *soft marketing*. Consumers generally do not respond well to hard selling, especially when they are in a position of perceived vulnerability, such as the dentist's chair. When you provide your patients with accurate information about a new service, you simultaneously create informed consumers and exert subtle marketing influence.

Strategies for Educating Staff to Educate Patients

You have several options when training your staff to serve as a well-informed, frontline marketing team for your niche practice:

- Many name brands, such as Invisalign, Cfast, Lumineers, or Whiter Image, provide training sessions specifically geared toward dental staff. These sessions generally include tips on marketing their products or services in addition to clinical training.
- If traveling to seminars or training sessions will not work well for your practice, online resources can be beneficial. Download and have your staff study clinical and marketing information about the new services you will offer.
- For each new service, dedicate a full staff meeting to discussing associated clinical basics, frequently asked questions, benefits or advantages, alternatives, and costs. Giving your staff the proper vocabulary with which to talk to patients about certain services will help them feel more at ease with performing the sales aspect of their job.
- Together with your front office staff, you may want to develop a phased payment plan or a simplified cost breakdown, so your staff can answer your patients' questions about cost.

Financing Options for Treatment

According to the American Dental Association, the number of Americans taking advantage of professional dental care has decreased 38.6 percent since 2007. A number of economic factors, including unemployment or underemployment and diminishing dental insurance benefits, contribute to this disheartening statistic.

To attract new patients to their niche practice even in times of economic uncertainty, business-savvy dentists provide their patients with a variety of financing and payment options. Letting your patients know you want to work with them to achieve the treatment they need shows you care about

them. Not only does this reinforce patient loyalty, but also, because specialists have a reputation for higher fees, your patients will be grateful that you
are able to perform more procedures yourself. It's a happy day all around
when the ability to finance procedures enables patients to move forward to
better health, function, comfort, and esthetics. If you manage your business
well, it will always be healthy for your practice bottom line.

When developing a financing plan for your new niche services, you will
need to evaluate your fees and consider payment and financing options for
patients.

Determining Fees

One cannot overstate the importance of determining the right fees for your
services before you begin treating patients. Basing your fee system on a solid
grasp of the time and materials needed to perform niche procedures requires
a realistic assessment of several factors:

- Time needed for you and your staff to perform the consultation, proce-
  dure, and follow-up care.
- Materials and equipment needed.
- Associated lab or shipping fees.
- National average cost of your service.
- Local average cost of your services.

How do the specific demographics of your area affect what you should
charge? For instance, the materials and time needed to place a veneer may be
consistent, but a dentist in a Houston suburb will not charge the same as a
dentist located in downtown Chicago.

Research the competition. If other dentists in your area offer a similar service, do you think you could charge more or less than the competition?

In-House Financing

In-house financing can provide a viable option in certain cases and in certain markets. However, this method of treatment financing can be prob-
lematic and work-intensive. First, you need the manpower to execute and
the financial ability to underwrite an unsecured loan to the patient. Second,
unless you have an established relationship with the patient and the patient
has a stellar track record of making payments, this option may not work for
your practice.

If you choose to implement in-house financing, then you will need a clearly defined collections strategy. Once the work has been performed, patients have little incentive to make the payments, and sending constant payment reminders can diminish their perception of your practice. On the other hand, patients tend to appreciate in-house financing since it offers them a safe, easy way to receive the care they need without having to put off treatment.

After determining fees, you can work with your payment coordinator to create a financing schedule. Most office accounting software programs such as QuickBooks or office management programs like Dentrix include a template for creating it. An in-house financed treatment plan might look like this:

> Dan has a cracked tooth, and you recommend placing a CEREC crown to save the tooth. With materials and service, the cost of placing that crown comes out to approximately $1,000. Dan makes an initial down payment of $200 and agrees that he will pay the remaining $800 in monthly installments over the next eighteen months. Instead of paying $1,000 out of pocket, Dan will pay just under $45 per month until the crown is paid off.

Again, before going forward with this option, you will need to seriously consider the extra work associated with offering in-house financing, specifically with payment notification and collection, and determine whether your existing staff can accommodate these changes.

Phased Treatment

A much better alternative to an in-house financing option is the phased treatment option. Similar in execution to in-house financing, a phased treatment plan allows patients to receive treatment in installments and take care of the fees at each stage of treatment before proceeding with the next one. This removes the need for your staff to deal with the collections and late payment notifications associated with in-house financing. Careful preparation on your part, as well as on the part of your payment coordinator, will yield a manageable plan that your patient will appreciate. A phased treatment plan might look like this:

> Jennifer wants to improve the appearance of her smile, and together you develop a smile makeover treatment plan that includes several procedures. You schedule the procedures to take place a few months apart, beginning with gum contouring on the two front teeth and followed by whitening, bonding to repair a chipped tooth, and

placing a veneer over a badly misshapen tooth. Jennifer pays for each procedure in full, and the time between procedures allows her to save for the next one. Over the course of several months, Jennifer achieves the smile she wants without putting a huge strain on her budget.

Third-Party Financing Options

If you have the right patient demographic (with a stable income and good credit scores), third-party financing is the best strategy to ensure stability of collections. After the money is collected, your two primary concerns are office production and efficient scheduling.

Teaming up with third-party financing companies takes two common forms:

- You can join a discount or referral plan. While you will have to discount your services, the increased volume of patients will likely make up for the income shortfall.
- Dental care credit companies such as CareCredit serve the same function as a credit card and offer your patients low-interest financing for a huge range of services. This option lets you receive your full payment up front.

If you think third-party financing might work well for your niche practice, set aside some time to adequately research the benefits and potential disadvantages for each option. You may want to consult with colleagues and see whether a local discount plan worked out for them. Scour message boards for feedback from patients and for specific, real-world examples of what works for different patients.

Incentives

Another way to increase interest in your new services is through financial incentives and other kinds of rewards.

Special Discounts and Promotions

Offering discounts, coupons, and special promotions for certain services or to certain patients is a proven way to increase business and drive your niche practice's profitability. Use the following list as a springboard for developing a plan for offering discounted fees:

- Provide one-time new-patient discounts on services, such as a complete exam and cleaning for a very low price, fifty dollars off teeth whitening, or a complimentary consultation for Six Month Smiles or Invisalign.
- Offer exclusive coupons for patients who "like" your business page on Facebook or who subscribe to your monthly newsletter.
- Offer a 5 to 10 percent discount for patients who prepay for their treatment.
- Look at your demographic research and determine whether offering a discount to certain groups might attract more business. For instance, if your practice is located near a military base, a large school district, or a senior living center, consider offering military, teacher, or senior discounts.

Smart Business Tip—*Be careful of using deep-discount promotions offered through online auction sites. Empirical studies have shown that deep discounts diminish the value of your services and most patients who sign up do not come back for additional treatment.*

Implementing Reward Systems

Providing staff incentives will help motivate your team to find opportunities to market your new niche services. Consider some of the following scenarios and how you might adapt them to the specific needs of your practice:

- You conduct free monthly lectures at the local community center about senior dental care and the advantages of implant-secured dentures. Offer an incentive for the staff member who signs up the most patients to attend each month's lecture.
- During a cleaning, your hygienist talks to a patient about Invisalign and the patient schedules a consultation with you. Whether or not the patient ultimately chooses Invisalign, your hygienist has successfully marketed the service and has earned a reward.
- Set monthly goals for certain services, such as in-office whitening treatments. If the team reaches that goal within the allotted time, everyone gets to enjoy a team reward.
- Post a chart with everyone's name and a roll of small stickers in the break room. Every time a staff member tries out a sales technique, whether the patient ultimately buys into the treatment or not, the staff member can place a sticker next to her or his name. Often, simple rewards are enough to motivate team members to dip their toes into the proverbial marketing pool.

The rewards you offer can vary from verbal recognition and a personal thank you to gift cards, tickets to a ball game or the movies, or an extended lunch break on Friday. Team rewards could be as simple as bringing in bagels and coffee to the next staff meeting. Learn what your staff values and tailor your rewards system to that.

Marketing Your Niche

Being able to touch so many people through my businesses and make money while doing it is a huge blessing.
—Magic Johnson

Branding Your Niche Practice

To understand the complex integration of marketing processes that make up brand development, it helps to consider that the end goal of successful niche practice branding occurs when you become the go-to dentist for a particular technique or service. Marketing tools that help grow your brand seek to achieve the following:

- Send a clear, informative message about your unique services that engages on an emotional and intellectual level.
- Attract prospective clients, inspire and secure their loyalty, and transform them into lifelong patients who will refer family and friends to your practice.
- Present you as the acknowledged local expert in a particular niche.

To help establish your niche brand, you will need to develop a dynamic marketing strategy that incorporates well-designed online resources, traditional print marketing such as newspaper ads, billboards, brochures, and business cards, and a visible presence in the community.

Online Marketing with Microsites—The New Trend in Niche Marketing

Microsites function exactly as their name implies. They are smaller, more condensed websites meant to promote only your niche services. A high-quality microsite complements your primary website but has a more simplified navigation, less content, and a sharper focus. Think about a microsite as your opportunity to distill your overall practice philosophy into a vibrant, concise message.

Of course, your microsite will also attract online attention through keyword optimization, tracking, and analytics. To help boost search engine ratings, many successful microsites link to a search-engine-friendly blog. Microsites are relatively inexpensive and easy to create, although unless you have particularly strong design and writing skills, you may want to engage a dental marketing firm to build your microsite for you.

Smart Business Tip—Be careful of relying on any single marketing strategy as the "silver bullet." Algorithm changes at Google and other search engines can quickly make your online strategy obsolete or irrelevant. Before engaging in microsites or blogs, focus on creating a great website full of original articles that clearly tell patients about you and inform them about what you offer and your expertise. Make sure the articles are well optimized and enticing so patients make that all-important phone call.

Social Networking

You have probably heard that social networking outlets such as Facebook and Twitter will help you market your practice. However, without a clear idea of how social networks can drive your brand development, you cannot successfully deploy them as part of your marketing strategy. Consider the three primary goals of an engaging and well-thought-out social-network marketing plan:

- First, social networking on its own can create buzz about your niche service, but linking to your microsite gives that buzz focus and purpose.
- Second, regular posting on your Facebook business page, blog, or Twitter account directs more traffic to your primary website, the cornerstone of your online marketing strategy.
- Finally, social media allows your loyal patients to make person-to-person recommendations with ease. By simply sharing your latest blog post or a link to your microsite, your existing patients have generated a prospect and helped establish you as an expert on a particular service.

Successful social media marketing depends on regularly updates with fresh content. Furthermore, different social networking sites offer distinct benefits for different practices. Consider the benefits of the four most well-known social networking venues.

Facebook—

Over half of people in the United States have Facebook pages and, contrary to popular belief, the median age of those users is thirty-three. This means that your primary customer base actively uses Facebook. This excellent social media tool allows you to link to your blog, microsite, or website. Through Facebook you can also offer exclusive promotions or giveaways to patients who have "liked" your page or posted pictures of you at the last big community event.

Twitter—

Twitter functions like a blog but in an extremely condensed format (140 characters and spaces or less). Posts to Twitter (called *tweets*) are indexed and can be easily searched through Google, Yahoo, Bing, and other search engines. Personalized Twitter accounts will help you grow your unique brand, run promotions, build local interest, and enhance your online presence.

YouTube—

YouTube videos serve several marketing functions. Keyword-rich titles, descriptions, and comments drive your search engine rankings higher. Informative videos also offer existing and prospective patients a means to learn about the procedures you offer and the materials you use. You can integrate your social media marketing by posting videos to Twitter and Facebook or by embedding them on your blog, microsite, or main website.

> **Smart Business Tip**—*Ignoring YouTube can be a serious impediment to your web marketing strategy in 2013 and beyond. Video has the ability to convert your lead into a patient who instantly calls your office after viewing a compelling presentation. According to Invodo. com, 51.9% of marketing professionals worldwide cite video as the type of content with the best ROI. Approximately half of marketers who use video in email campaigns see increased click-through rates, increased time spent reading the email, and increased sharing and forwarding*

Blogs—

Most people use blogs as a source for trustworthy information on a specific topic. Fresh, original, keyword-rich content will drive your blog higher in search engine results pages. Linking your blog to your website or microsite gives prospective patients a direct route to information about your niche practice. Sites such as WordPress offer users a free, easy-to-use format for starting a blog. However, unless you or a staff member have highly developed writing skills, you may want to work with a reputable and accountable dental marketing firm and have them write high-quality informative content.

Depending on the makeup of your staff, you have several options for handling your practice's social marketing strategy. You could assign it to a front office staff member or office coordinator. If you feel that you have the communication skills necessary to post well-worded content, you can even take over the job yourself. There are a few reputable dental marketing firms or consultants who have the experience and skill to deploy your social network marketing campaign so it yields the best outcomes.

> *Smart Business Tip—Choose your marketing experts wisely. Most dental marketing companies offer fragmented solutions that focus on only a few aspects of marketing strategy. Most stand-alone strategies like search engine optimization (SEO), search engine marketing (SEM), and social media fail because they are not integrated with your overall strategic marketing goals. Accountability is something you must demand from every expert you hire.*

Today's Word of Mouth;

When it comes to marketing, nothing beats word of mouth or its viral equivalent. Marketing experts assert that word-of-mouth recommendations drive business because people innately trust the opinions of people with whom they have a personal relationship. Word-of-mouth marketing depends heavily on the quality of clinical care and customer service you provide in the office. Exceptional service that exceeds patient expectations will prompt personal recommendations. Other strategies for generating word-of-mouth endorsements include establishing a positive community presence.

Although they take place in the somewhat impersonal environment of online communication, word-of-mouth referrals can generate website and microsite traffic and move your niche practice forward. Today, word of mouth takes many forms, including online reviews, links or blogs shared on Facebook, and forwarded newsletters or e-blasts.

Social media—

Make the most of social media:

- Run exclusive promotions and giveaways (such as a 50 percent coupon for teeth whitening or a free sonic toothbrush) for people who "like" your Facebook page or follow you on Twitter.
- Respond to comments and questions on Facebook, Twitter, YouTube, and your blog. Quick responses let people know you care and want to engage and help them on a personal level.
- Share the latest news in your field that consumers may want to read and share with their friends. This serves two purposes. It positions you as an expert on the cutting edge of your profession and also keeps you front and center in your patients' minds. An office manager can be easily trained for this weekly routine.

Testimonials—

Ask for testimonials and post them to your website, microsite, blog, and other social media outlets. Some successful dentists even video their patients' testimonials and post the videos online. However, before asking a patient for a testimonial, check with your state dental association's advertising guidelines to see if posting testimonials is an allowable practice.

Begin with your friends, family, and staff (and their friends and family) and encourage them to:

- Make positive personal recommendations.
- "Like" your Facebook page, follow you on Twitter, or subscribe to your YouTube channel.
- Organize a limited-time special offer that donates a dollar to a local charity for every "like" you get for your business page. Your friends will feel great about themselves for doing a good deed, and you will get great visibility.
- Write online reviews on websites such as Doctoroogle, Yelp, or Angie's List.

Reputation—

Monitor your reputation by checking on your online marketing outlets frequently. If someone leaves a negative comment on your latest Facebook post, it can leave a bad impression with potential clients if you do not respond. Your response should create a positive spin, offer your apologies, and demonstrate your dedication to resolving issues quickly.

__Smart Business Tip__—Reputation is truly the currency of business today, especially if you are offering a service. Without a stellar reputation, your practice stands no chance of competing against savvier dentists who have figured out a way to harness the power of reputation for their own good.

Print Marketing

While print news media may struggle in today's digitally driven world, print advertising continues to thrive. Print marketing tools such as business cards, informative brochures, billboards, and newspaper or magazine ads make up an essential aspect of a well-rounded marketing strategy by offering:

Permanence and portability—

When prospective patients walk away from your expo booth, free lecture, or in-office consultation with a business card or brochure, they have a physical artifact to keep their interaction with you fresh.

Prestige—

Many people, especially those who did not grow up steeped in Internet culture, prefer print to online media. This is especially true in the older demographic—pen and paper still dominate over keyboard and mouse.

Professional design—

Although you may be tempted to design your own business cards and promotional items, the results may not give the polished, professional, brand-reinforcing impression you want. We strongly encourage you to work closely with a professional marketing firm with industry experience to help create visually engaging, informative, and easy-to-understand print marketing tools that are highly targeted to existing and new patients.

Direct Mail

In addition to handouts and print "collateral," targeted direct mail is a force to be reckoned with. The reason is simple. The combination of print and direct mail gives you a surefire way to put your advertisement in the hands of the customer or prospect on a specific day. No form or digital media can do that. Moreover, high-impact pieces like tri-fold or barrel-fold brochures convey more information in a compact manner. Magnets and magnet postcards can create tangible value for consumers and offer a daily reminder of your services when they reach into the refrigerator.

The return on investment on surgically targeted postcard campaigns has shown surprisingly tremendous promise in many important industries including pizza restaurants, automobiles, sports, and believe it or not, dentistry. Through precise targeting and data modeling you can compile a list of ideal patients and focus your efforts on them by delivering a high-impact direct mail piece. Finding the right partner, who has capabilities in variable imaging and exact in-home dates, is crucial.

Local Publicity

Like the fire station, the corner store, and the post office, a dental practice occupies a place of prestige within any given community. This built-in cachet allows most dentists to transition into becoming outstanding community supporters and leaders with relative ease. Seeking out service projects, supporting local advertising outlets, and otherwise creating a positive impact in your community serves two functions. It gives you a sense of purpose and it increases your practice's visibility. Use the following list of ideas as a springboard for enhancing your niche practice marketing strategy:

- Utilize local advertising outlets.
- Sponsor a youth sports team.
- Take out an advertisement in the high school musical program.
- Contribute to the monthly community newsletter.
- Team up with a local charity and volunteer your time or consider sponsoring an event, such as a 5K run or fall festival.

- Set up a booth at the next bridal exposition and offer free cosmetic consultations for prospective brides.
- Volunteer your services by giving free checkups or hosting a lecture at a community health fair.

Every community differs from the next, so you will need to put some research into what publicity opportunities are available. How you choose to publicize your niche practice locally should depend upon the demographic information you have compiled.

Chapter Three:
Gauging Success

The only limits are, as always, those of vision.
–James Broughton

Setting Realistic Goals

Winning is not a sometime thing; it's an all time thing.
You don't win once in a while, you don't do things right once in a while, you
do them right all the time. Winning is habit. Unfortunately, so is losing.
—Vince Lombardi

Defining Success

Only you can determine how you will assess the success of your niche practice. Of course, the bottom-line profitability of your practice—how much you take home at the end of the day—plays a large role in gauging your success. How quickly you rolled out your niche services and how much revision those services required factor into the practice's success. Other, less-tangible measures also play a huge role in figuring out how successful your expanded practice is. To help outline your unique idea of success, you should ask yourself the following questions:

What do you want your practice to look like in ten years?

- Do you want to serve a high volume of patients?
- Do you want to offer a wide range of services, acting as a one-stop dental practice with an in-house prosthetics lab or staff anesthesiologist?
- Do you want to become a boutique dental practice, offering the very best of just a few services to a lower volume of patients?

How do you envision yourself in ten years?

You are the most integral part of your practice. Personal development goes hand in hand with professional development, so make sure to have a clear idea where you want this new niche to take you.

- Do you want to be a respected lecturer or teach classes at the nearby dental school?
- Do you want to write a book or become a regular contributor to a respected dentistry website?
- Do you want to become a more active member, or even take on a leadership role, in a professional dental association?

Write it down.

Take fifteen to thirty minutes to sit and brainstorm how you envision your successful niche practice. Use the notes you take during this session to create a formalized map to success, with clearly defined steps. Revisit the map at regular intervals to see how your actual progress corresponds to your projections.

Evaluating Expenses

Before going forward with a plan for expanding your practice, you will need to perform a comprehensive expense evaluation of your current practice. You will need to consider a huge range of factors including rent, utilities, equipment leasing and maintenance, office supplies, clinical materials, employee salary and benefits, insurance, code compliance and licenses, and waste management.

While you should absolutely have a clear idea of the expenses associated with the day-to-day operation of your practice, accurate expense evaluations are best performed by a professional accountant with experience in small business and dental or medical practices. Dental CPAs have the skill and time needed to thoroughly assess your expenses and make the best recommendations for where to direct your practice.

A Realistic Timeline

To determine a realistic timeline for debuting your niche services, break the total time needed into three phases.

1) ***Planning, research, and analysis***—This includes market research, demographic research, product and equipment research, space planning, and expense and budget analysis.

2) ***Training***—Get a clear idea of how much time you and your staff will need to dedicate to familiarizing yourselves with equipment and procedures. Some

niche services, such as teeth whitening or sleep apnea treatment, may not require as much training as the more complex procedures such as surgical tooth extractions.

3) *Implementation*—This includes ordering, shipping, and setting up equipment, gathering and inventorying the necessary tools and materials, marketing, and advertising.

Evaluation and Revision

The time you spend preparing to debut your niche practice is relatively short compared to the time you will spend honing your skills and refining the day-to-day operation of your office. After you begin offering your new services to patients, build on your existing timeline and schedule yearly or twice-yearly practice evaluations to determine whether your practice is moving in the direction you envisioned. Consider the following five areas of evaluation:

1) *Finances*—You will need your accountant to assess your finances and determine whether your niche services are paying for themselves. He or she can also help you locate areas where streamlining a process may help you cut down on overhead costs.

2) *Refining your skills*—Do you feel that your skill level is improving? Do you feel more comfortable performing a procedure now than when the service debuted? Have you read about a new technique or material that you would like to give a try? Look into continuing education opportunities if you feel that you are ready to continue developing your clinical skill.

3) *Customer satisfaction*—Using online, print, or person-to-person survey techniques, get a feel for how your patients are responding to your expanded services. If areas of dissatisfaction exist, how can you alter your process to accommodate change?

4) *Staff satisfaction*—How does your hygiene staff feel about the new services? Do they feel they require more training or more assistance from you in any way? Does your front office staff feel that patients are responding positively to fees and payment plans? What kinds of frontline response are they receiving from patients?

5) *Self-check*—Do you enjoy providing these new services? Do you feel that they are pushing your practice toward your ten-year goal? Have you noticed that you have an aptitude for a certain procedure and want to explore further

developing that aspect of your practice? For instance, you may have begun offering several cosmetic treatments, but you notice you have a knack with veneers. Would becoming the local veneers expert be in line with your plan for personal and professional success?

Expanding Your Niche

To be successful, you have to have your heart in your business, and your business in your heart.
—Thomas Watson, Sr.

A dental practice, much like any other small business, is always a work in progress. Technology, best practices, notions of beauty, health, and sustainability, the demographics of your client base, and patient demands change constantly. You have to adapt your practice to meet these changes. Staying informed and aware will allow you to identify points of improvement or progress that could help you expand your niche. Some of these techniques will help you stay ahead of the curve:

Journals

Subscribe to professional journals. Many professional organizations, such as the American Dental Association and the American Academy of Cosmetic Dentistry, provide free print and online subscriptions for members. Peer-reviewed journals offer dentists the very latest research on techniques, technology, materials, and trends particular to your niche.

Two-Way Communication

Maintain consistent two-way communication between you and your staff. Often, dentists have a more circumspect, big-picture view of a practice, while staff members tend to have a more detail-oriented view. Communication helps dentists and their staff unify their views for a more complete understanding of the practice.

Your Dental CPA

Enlist the help of your dental CPA. A professional dental CPA has the tools and know-how to look at your finances and identify areas in need of improvement. He or she can also make informed recommendations for streamlining your finances and boosting your bottom line. When you choose a CPA, make sure the CPA understands not just accounting and taxes, but your specific industry, that is, dentistry. CPA firms who specialize in serving dentists are able to provide you with real-world insights that can help you make good decisions and prevent you from making bad ones. My own firm, Reliance Consulting LLC (www.reliancecpa.com), has been advising dentists since 1984 and continues to lead the way in helping dentists achieve their financial goals.

Dental Practice Consultants

If you feel that your niche practice has stalled, profits have slipped, or the day-to-day operations don't run as smoothly as they should, you may want to bring in a consultant. Dental marketing and practice consultants have a great deal of experience working with all kinds of dental practices, helping them streamline office operations and kick-start their forward momentum. Often, simply bringing in a third-party expert can provide the objective perspective needed to identify problems. Dental consultants can perform a wide range of services, including:

- Evaluating the effectiveness of your current marketing strategy and offering suggestions for revision.
- Reviewing and refining the goals you initially determined when you debuted your niche services.
- Streamlining operations such as patient paperwork, coding, patient flow, accounts receivable procedures, scheduling practices, and more.
- Helping you develop the skills you need to act as the leader of your practice, including personnel techniques, hiring and termination practices, and developing attractive benefits packages.

Even if you feel as though your niche practice has reached the highest possible level of success and you are enjoying steady profits, a consistent patient base, and a great deal of professional satisfaction, you should never stop asking, "Is there anything I can do to make this better?"

Smart Business Tip—*Without a continuous improvement (CI) mindset, Toyota would have never reached the pinnacle of the automobile world. If Apple was satisfied with the iPod and had not embraced CI, the iPhone would not be a reality today.*

Chapter Four:
Resources

As you begin the research and planning phase of developing your niche practice, we encourage you to delve into the vast online resources provided by professional dental associations. These websites provide you with the best source for accurate, up-to-date information that will guide your decision-making process. Furthermore, most offer article libraries, surveys, and advice for dentists wanting to expand their general practices.

Recommended Websites

Academy of General Dentistry

The AGD (www.agd.org) offers a good starting point for general dentists wanting to expand into the niche practice market. Active member forums yield lots of tips and advice based on real-life experience. You can also access the article library of *General Dentistry*, the AGD's peer-reviewed journal.

Academy of Laser Dentistry

If you think laser dentistry might be the right niche for you, the ALD (www.laserdentistry.org) offers a wealth of information, advice, training and continuing education opportunities, active member forums, and information about vendors and federal regulations. You and your staff can also earn certifications through the ALD.

American Academy of Cosmetic Dentistry

A highly regarded professional dental organization, the AACD (www.aacd.com) is dedicated to the advancement of ethical, scientifically sound, and, above all, esthetic cosmetic dentistry practices. Through the AACD, general dentists interested in developing a cosmetic niche can find resources for accreditation, a huge selection of webinars, eLearning opportunities, and conferences, vendor information, and charitable opportunities. The *Journal of Cosmetic Dentistry*, the AACD's peer-reviewed publication, provides the most current research on a wide range of cosmetic dental techniques, materials, and issues.

American Academy of Dental Sleep Medicine

For general dentists who want to learn more about snoring and sleep apnea treatment, the AADSM (www.aadsm.org) offers many resources to help them get started. To fulfill their mission of promoting the dentist's role in treating snoring and sleep apnea through the use of oral appliance therapy, the AADSM provides:

- A variety of educational opportunities for every level of experience.
- Online and dentist-to-dentist networking opportunities.
- Tips for successfully collaborating with medical sleep specialists.
- Advice and toolkits for marketing your sleep apnea and snoring treatment niche.
- Access to the very latest research and innovation through *Sleep and Breathing*, the AADSM's peer-reviewed journal.

American Academy of Implant Dentistry

The AAID (www.aaid-implant.org) is the go-to resource for information about all phases of dental implant placement. Through the AAID, you can access a wealth of educational materials including seminars, training courses, webinars, eLearning platforms, active member forums, and DVD training series. You can also locate industry news and, should you decide that you want to expand your dental implant niche to include both phases of placement, the AAID offers educational and accreditation opportunities.

American Association of Endodontists

Even if you do not want to formally specialize in endodontics, the AAE (www.aae.org) provides a vast amount of information and several educational opportunities for general dentists wishing to augment their skills so they can expand their practice. Resources include:

- Original podcasts
- Article and press release libraries
- Product and vendor directories

- Toolkits for public relations and marketing
- Glossaries, annual reports, and links to further resources

American Association of Orthodontics

Much of the information you need for expanding into accelerated orthodontics services will depend on which brands you choose to offer. A wealth of professional reviews of various orthodontic systems can be found on http://www.aaomembers.org/resources/index.cfm. Can't decide whether you want to offer Invisalign or ClearCorrect? Searching the AAO's article libraries will yield a great deal of helpful information.

American Dental Association

The gold standard of dental professional resources, the ADA (http://www.ada.org/professional.aspx) offers everything from continuing education opportunities and licensure to product directories and business resources. The ADA also boasts a treasure trove of information for developing, managing, and growing your niche practice. The ADA can also help you stay at the cutting edge of research, no matter your niche, through its journals, the *Journal of the American Dental Association* and *Evidence-Based Dentistry*.

CEREC Online

CEREC Impression and Chairside CAD/CAM Solutions are offered by Sirona Dental Systems. Should you decide that CEREC might be the right direction for your niche practice, CEREC Online (www.cereconline.com) provides a wealth of educational and training opportunities, FAQs, member forums, and support.

International Congress of Oral Implantologists—Implant Prosthetics Section

This international organization offers many of the same resources as the AAID. However, the ICOI (icoi.org/implant-prosthetics-section.php) also offers focused training and education in implant prosthetics or restorations.

Reliance Consulting LLC

Reliance Consulting LLC (www.reliancecpa.com) offers customized tax, accounting, and business consulting services to dentists nationwide. From automating the accounting and payroll systems to bill pay and tax services, Reliance also offers guidance in the areas of practice valuation, practice growth, retirement planning, estate planning, and asset protection. The CPAs and consultants at Reliance are well versed in dentistry and can provide you with highly customized solutions. The author of this book is the managing partner of Reliance.

Dentist Profit Systems LLC

Dentist Profit Systems LLC (www.dentistprofitsystems.com) was cofounded by the author of this book in response to growing popularity and the success he had with consulting clients in marketing strategy, both online and offline. Dentist Profit Systems has developed a unique DR.4 system for practice growth and profitability. (See *Marketing Epilogue* below.)

Marketing Epilogue

Building Accountable Marketing Systems

Think of planning, preparation, marketing, and development of your niche special services as analogous to the diagnosis, treatment planning, treatment, and optimal refinement of a patient's oral health, function, and esthetics. You would not allow a nondentist to diagnose, treatment plan, and treat your mouth. You are likely wondering how you—a dentist, albeit a business owner—can be expected to evaluate your local market, market your new services, and grow your patient base for these services in a professional and profitable manner.

A Google search for dental marketing today yields 32.7 million results. In today's marketplace, there is an abundance of dental marketing experts who promise you everything from improved search engine rankings to super fancy social media campaigns to bright, shiny websites. Words like SEO, SEM, social media, and mobile strategy have become so ubiquitous that most dentists believe having any or all of the buzzwords will automatically translate into new patients. Fancy website design that automatically responds to mobile devices seems to be the latest marketing gimmick being touted as a panacea capable of harnessing the power of an increasingly mobile populace.

Many companies, in an effort to win over less-informed audiences, showcase complex Google algorithms and whiteboards replete with flowcharts, implicitly indicating technical prowess. This technical prowess is expected to magically translate into hundreds of new patients and astronomical dental profits.

The luxury of being a managing partner of a CPA firm with eight hundred corporate clients is that it allows you tremendous insight into the workings of all business. From corporate strategy and tax optimization to asset protection and marketing strategy, no topic is off-limits. Creating value from effective decision making has been the hallmark of our CPA practice, and clients from all over the country have sought our advice in helping optimize their business operations.

My own experiments with client acquisition over the past four years taught me valuable lessons on the pitfalls of one-size-fits-all strategies. The marketing techniques we employed over these four years have yielded tremendous results and contributed to the quality growth of our accounting practice.

The research in writing this book, coupled with my own experience at Reliance Consulting, helped me conceptualize and create a new accountable concept in dental marketing. It's called *Dentist Profit Systems*. It's a time-tested approach that goes back to the fundamentals of marketing strategy and leverages today's technology to deliver superior accountable results.

There is no industry jargon to tout or fancy algorithms to showcase. It's a simple model that looks at the four most important aspects of marketing for dental practice success. Those four aspects are enshrined in our *DR.4* system, which takes Marketing 101 and supercharges it in today's environment.

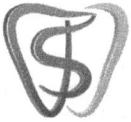

Dentist Profit Systems

Dentist Profit Systems (DPS) offers a unique combination of services to guide you and assist you with each step of the planning, preparation, assessment, and expansion of your niche practice, as outlined in this book. You are invited to take a look at http://www.dentistprofitsystems.com and learn about the DR.4 system of processes for:

- Dentist Reach Enhancement
- Dentist Reputation Builder
- Dentist Reengagement
- Dentist Referral Optimization

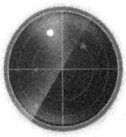

DPS: Dentist Reach Enhancement

Before we begin your optimization services, we learn a lot about you and your local community. Together, we discover not only what you want to do more of, but also what your community members want. Is your community full of young families, replete with near-retirement communities, or is it in a cosmopolitan area? Is there a sizable market share searching for family dentistry? Are there many older citizens searching for dental implant expertise? Is there a large population of adults seeking clear orthodontics or cosmetic procedures like teeth whitening and veneers? We determine the keywords they search.

We then reach out to your potential new clients with a well-designed mobile website, keyword ads, and unique web content that is matched to what they are seeking. Because stories naturally compel humans to become engaged, we will include videos that showcase these sought-after services. And, because patients want to be informed, trust in your expertise, and know you genuinely care about what is in their best interest, your campaign will include custom blog posts and expert articles on your areas of expertise. Everything we do will be visually tied together with custom branding graphics designed specifically for your practice.

One of the ways DR.4 differs from other dentist marketing programs is in our customization of videos for your website. These videos focus on your specialties, tour your facility, and provide video press releases, patient testimonials, and informational video brochures. Your custom network of videos will show up on your website and through broader syndication to ensure you communicate in a highly effective way.

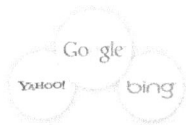

DPS: Dentist Reputation Builder

Our DR.4 services not only include custom videos and articles to position you as an expert, but also offer you a digital tablet-based kiosk that patients can use to write reviews before leaving your office. Your staff will be trained to respond to this feedback immediately, alert you if a negative experience needs to be addressed, take steps to harness the power of positive feedback, and share the input socially to extend your reach to new business.

You already know the *why*. We will teach you what, when, and how to collect and leverage reviews using the latest digital technologies and most popular social media. A proven tracking system is included to help you continuously enhance the patient experience and build lifelong successes with your clients.

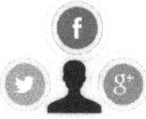

DPS: Dentist Reengagement

After clients leave, it's critical that you continue to make them feel cared for. This includes more than a follow-up postcard; it encompasses using e-mail, media, and social media to keep your client base continuously engaged. Our services offer not only coaching in this essential area but also the option of custom-written e-mail templates, news, postcards, and frequent social media posts.

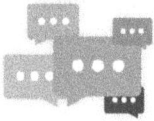

DPS: Dentist Referral Optimization

Finally, we believe that word-of-mouth references are among the strongest marketing tools available. Most dental practices have yet to make use of social media, on-hold messaging, and incentive contests to engage existing and new patients. We provide a host of methods, including those just mentioned, to generate word-of-mouth stories and praise both online and in-person. We make it easy for your current clients to share their experiences with others who might very well be your next clients.

Free Consultation

Our services have been tested by real practices in a wide variety of geographic and demographic settings. The results have been amazing—analyzing what local patients are looking for, generating top search engine placement for those qualities, producing steady growth in new patient phone calls, creating better informed and trusting patients, improving case acceptance, increasing profitability, increasing patient satisfaction, and making a more confident staff and happier dentists.

Our DR.4 services are designed to effectively take your practice to the people you want to reach and engage as new clients, build your reputation, and establish a system that will keep you engaged with your clients and secure their loyalty and referrals.

At DPS, we rely on measurable, reputation-based activities that drive lifelong patients and revenue:

- Social media-style reputation building
- Creative referral opportunities
- Targeted patient care follow-up
- In-office feedback kiosks
- Evaluation of the patient experience
- Cost tracking for new patient acquisitions
- Custom thought leadership content
- Mobile marketing solutions

For a free consultation about your practice needs, please contact the author at amol@dentistprofitsystems.com or visit www.dentistprofitsystems.com.

About the Author

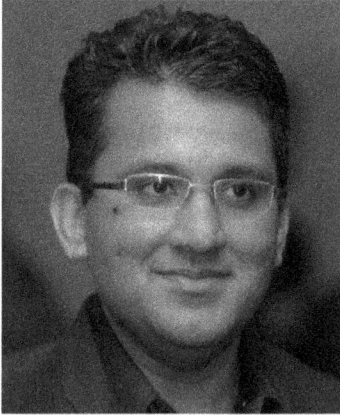

Amol Nirgudkar, CPA, CGMA

Amol graduated top of his class from the University of South Florida and obtained a bachelor of science in finance, a bachelor of science in accounting, and a master of science in accounting. He obtained his CPA certification thereafter and has been in public accounting for over thirteen years.

Amol serves as the CEO of Reliance Consulting LLC and Dentist Profit Systems LLC. He brings a tremendous wealth of knowledge and experience as a CPA and business advisor to hundreds of small businesses across Florida and the United States.

Throughout his professional career as a CPA, Amol has advised clients ranging from small businesses to large corporations and provided sophisticated tax and advisory services.

Over the last decade, Amol has developed a significant niche in the healthcare space and has served over five hundred physicians and over one hundred dentists in the Florida market.

In addition to publishing several articles on topics ranging from taxation to healthcare, he has authored a handbook, *Navigating the Business of Medicine*, for medical residents and physicians who wish to start their own private practice.

Amol has helped evolve Reliance Consulting from a tax and accounting firm into a business-consulting practice that helps small businesses with corporate strategy, marketing strategy, and innovation. In his view, without innovation, it is difficult for businesses to survive and thrive in today's economy. Amol has advised and helped many organizations with innovative strategies that are essential to succeed in today's complex environment.

Reliance Consulting LLC stands out as a unique value proposition within the CPA firm marketplace. From tax strategy and navigating the complex and dynamic regulations to consulting with businesses, Amol has pioneered the concept of "total business transformation" to achieve strategic goals, through innovation.

Dentist Profit Systems LLC, under Amol's leadership, aims to create a sophisticated and holistic dental marketing system that addresses all aspects of patient acquisition, retention, and referral. Using the latest online and offline tools and combining them with in-house practice optimization through training and consulting programs, the team at Dentist Profit Systems is dedicated to building truly great dental practices from the inside out.